Table of Contents

A colonoscopy is an outpatient procedure that is done to examine the inside of your large intestine (colon and rectum). The examination uses an instrument called a colonoscope (sometimes called a scope). This flexible instrument is very long and includes a camera and the ability to remove tissue (you won't feel the tissue being removed). A colonoscopy is commonly used to evaluate gastrointestinal symptoms, such as bleeding, abdominal pain or changes in bowel habits (how often you poop, how easily you poop, and the color and consistency of your poop).

BREAKFAST

1. Pumpkin Fluff

Prep Time: 10 Minutes

Cook Time: 30 Minutes

Servings: 5

Ingredients

- 1 cup cream cheese (8 oz.) - softened
- ¾ cup brown sugar
- ½ cup pure pumpkin purée
- ¾ teaspoon pumpkin pie spice
- ½ cup heavy cream
- Garnishes:
- Cinnamon powder
- Lotus Biscoff cookies - crumbled

Instructions

1. In a medium bowl with an electric hand mixer on medium speed, beat the cream cheese and brown sugar together.
2. 1 cup cream cheese (8 oz.), ¾ cup brown sugar
3. Add the pumpkin purée and pumpkin pie spice and combine until smooth.
4. ½ cup pure pumpkin purée, ¾ teaspoon pumpkin pie spice
5. In a separate bowl, whip the heavy cream with an electric hand mixer, until stiff peaks form (about 3 to 4 minutes).
6. ½ cup heavy cream
7. Gently fold the whipped cream into the cream cheese mixture with a spatula.
8. Refrigerate for 30 minutes or more.
9. Garnish with the cinnamon and crumbled Biscoff cookies. Serve with your favorite fruit, biscuits, graham crackers, etc.

Prep Time: 10 Minutes

Cook Time: 20 Minutes

Servings: 4

Ingredients

- 2 tbsp. olive oil
- 4 Yukon Gold potatoes - cubed
- 1 tsp. salt - or to taste
- ½ tsp. pepper - or to taste
- 1 white or yellow onion - chopped
- 5 Italian sausages - casings removed
- 1 red bell pepper - chopped
- 1 cup green onions - chopped
- 4 eggs
- Pink Himalayan salt
- Fresh parsley - chopped

Instructions

1. Heat an electric skillet to 300°F and add the olive oil.

2. Add the cubed potatoes. Season with the salt and pepper. Give it a mix so that the potatoes are coated in the oil. Cover and cook for 6 minutes, stirring occasionally.

3. Add the onions. Cover and cook for another 3 minutes, stirring occasionally.

4. Crumble the sausages into the pan. Add the red bell pepper and green onions and stir.

5. Reduce the heat to 250°F. Cover and continue cooking until the sausage and potatoes are cooked through (the potatoes should be fork-tender), another 10 minutes or so. Mix every few minutes.

6. Taste for seasoning and adjust with salt and pepper, if needed. Reserve.

7. Turn the heat up to 275°F. Fry the eggs until desired doneness.

8. Serve the eggs on top of the potatoes. Sprinkle with Himalayan salt and chopped parsley.

Prep Time: 15 Minutes

Cook Time: 8 Minutes

Servings: 4

Ingredients

For the Porridge Base:

- 1 ½ cups quick oats
- 1 cup milk
- 2 cups water
- ¼ cup sugar - or sugar substitute
- ¼ tsp. salt

Toppings:

- Strawberry slices, yogurt and poppy seeds
- Peanut butter, jelly and chopped hazelnuts
- Banana slices, maple syrup and cinnamon
- Jellies, crushed sweet biscuits (like graham wafers) and mini chocolate chips - (you could use mini marshmallows instead of jellies for a s'mores version!)

Instructions

1. Combine rolled oats, milk and water in a medium saucepan.
2. Add sugar and salt. Mix well. Bring to a boil.
3. Lower heat to a simmer. Cook (uncovered) until creamy and oats are softened, about 3 to 5 minutes, stirring occasionally. Remove from heat, cover and let ret rest for around 2 minutes.
4. Spoon the porridge into 8 (4 oz.) shot glasses or small jars, leaving some room for the toppings.
5. Serve the porridge shots with the topping options above (or use your kids' favorite toppings!). There will be 2 shot glasses for each porridge topping. Kids can pick and choose their porridge. This is a fun way to get kids to eat their breakfast!

Prep Time: 10 Minutes

Cook Time: 15 Minutes

Servings: 16

Ingredients

- 1 stick salted butter softened
- ¼ cup light brown sugar packed
- ¼ cup granulated sugar
- 1 tablespoon ground cinnamon
- 1 teaspoon vanilla extract
- 2 cans crescent rolls

For the glaze:

- 2 cups powdered sugar
- 3-4 tablespoons milk
- 2 teaspoons vanilla extract

Instructions

1. Preheat the oven to 375°F. Line sheet trays with parchment paper, set aside.

2. Place the softened butter, brown sugar, granulated sugar, cinnamon, and vanilla into a medium-sized bowl. Mix with an electric hand mixer until combined and smooth.

3. Unroll the crescent rolls and lay them on a clean work surface.

4. Spread a scant tablespoon of the filling over the dough.

5. Roll into a crescent shape and tuck the pointy ends under. Place on a prepared sheet tray about 3 inches apart. Repeat with the remaining rolls.

6. Bake for 11-13 minutes until golden brown on top. Some of the filling will escape while baking.

7. While the rolls are baking, make the glaze by whisking the powdered sugar, 3 tablespoons of the milk, and the vanilla into a shallow bowl. If it seems too thick, add up to another tablespoon of milk to reach the desired consistency. It should be thick yet pourable.

8. Allow the rolls to cool slightly. Dip the tops of the rolls one by one into the glaze, allowing any excess to drip off.

9. Place them glaze side up onto a wire rack over a sheet tray to catch any drips. Repeat with the remaining rolls.

10. Wait 15-30 minutes to allow the glaze to harden and serve immediately.

Prep Time: 10 Minutes

Cook Time: 15 Minutes

Servings: 4

Ingredients

- French Toast Sticks:
- 8 slices bread day-old
- 6-7 tablespoons Nutella
- 3 medium eggs
- ⅓ cup whole milk or almond, oat, coconut milk
- 1 teaspoon vanilla extract
- 2 tablespoons butter
- Coating:
- 4 tablespoons granulated sugar
- 1 ½ teaspoon ground cinnamon

Instructions

1. Lay out your bread slices and cut the crusts off.

2. Spread Nutella on a bread slice and add another slice on top to make a sandwich. Repeat with the remaining bread slices.
3. Cut each sandwich lengthwise, into 3 thick pieces and set them aside.
4. In a shallow dish, add eggs, milk and vanilla and mix well.
5. In a separate shallow dish combine cinnamon and sugar, set aside.
6. Melt butter in a large pan over medium high heat.
7. Once the butter is melted, dip each stick in the egg mixture (don't soak).
8. Place in the pan, and cook in batches until they're golden brown on each side.
9. Use tongs to transfer sticks in the cinnamon mixture and roll to coat all sides with the sweet mixture.
10. Serve immediately with Nutella, maple syrup or honey for dipping.

Prep Time: 20 Minutes

Cook Time: 20 Minutes

Servings: 6

Ingredients

For the crust:

- 2 ½ cups all-purpose flour
- 2 tablespoons granulated sugar
- 1 cup cold salted butter cut into cubes
- 1 teaspoon vanilla extract
- ½ cup cold water

For the filling:

- ½ cup light brown sugar packed
- 1 tablespoon salted butter melted
- 1 tablespoon all-purpose flour
- 2 teaspoons ground cinnamon

For the glaze:

- 1 cup powdered sugar
- ½ teaspoon ground cinnamon

- 1-2 tablespoons whole milk
- ½ teaspoon vanilla extract

Instructions

1. Place the flour and sugar into a food processor. Pulse a few times to combine.
2. Add the cold cubed butter and pulse until combined, the butter should be broken up and there should be no butter pieces larger than a pea.
3. Add the vanilla. Slowly stream in the water while the food processor is running. You want the crust to just come together, do not overmix.
4. Form the crust into a ball and cover with plastic wrap. Place in the refrigerator for 20-30 minutes to chill.
5. Preheat the oven to 400°F. Line a large sheet tray with parchment paper, and set it aside.
6. Make the filling by stirring together the brown sugar, butter, flour, and cinnamon until fully combined and set aside.
7. On a lightly floured clean work surface, roll out the dough into a 1/4th inch thick rough rectangle shape.
8. Using a 3x4 inch rectangle cookie cutter or something of similar size, cut out rectangles from the dough. You

will need to roll out the scraps of dough again to cut more rectangles. We need 12 pieces.

9. Place 6 of the crusts onto the prepared sheet tray, not touching.

10. Place just under 2 tablespoons of the filling into the center of each crust with a ¼ inch border.

11. Top with another crust and gently press down the edges. Take a fork and press the edges together to seal. Take the same fork and make 6 rows of ventilation holes over the center of the tarts.

12. Bake for 15-18 minutes until golden brown. Let cool completely.

13. For the glaze, whisk together the powdered sugar, cinnamon, milk, and vanilla extract. We want the glaze very thick but still pourable. Start with 1 tablespoon of the milk and add a little more at a time until the desired consistency.

14. Place the tarts onto a wire rack over a sheet tray to catch any drips. Spoon the glaze on top of the tarts. Let the glaze set for 20 minutes.

Prep Time: 15 Minutes

Cook Time: 25 Minutes

Servings: 12

Ingredients

- 1 ½ cups all-purpose flour
- 2 teaspoon baking powder
- 1 teaspoon fine sea salt
- ½ teaspoon ground cinnamon
- ½ cup vegetable oil
- ¾ cup light brown sugar packed
- 2 large eggs
- ½ cup sour cream
- 1 tablespoon vanilla extract
- 2 tablespoons whole milk
- 1 ¼ cups small chopped peeled fresh peaches

For the streusel:

- 6 tablespoons granulated sugar
- 4 tablespoons unsalted butter melted
- ⅔ cup all-purpose flour

- ½ teaspoon fine sea salt

Instructions

1. Preheat the oven to 425°F and line a 12-count muffin tin with paper liners, or spray them with baking spray before setting the tin aside.
2. Stir together the flour, baking powder, salt, and cinnamon in a medium mixing bowl, set aside.
3. Whisk together the oil and sugar until combined, in a large mixing bowl.
4. Add the eggs into the wet ingredients and whisk until smooth.
5. Then, add the sour cream and vanilla, and whisk until smooth.
6. Next, add the dry ingredient mixture to the wet ingredients and stir them together until they're just combined, with no dry patches.
7. Then, add in the milk to the batter and stir until well incorporated.
8. Add the chopped peaches to the batter and fold them in.
9. Divide and pour the batter among the 12 muffin sections, set aside.

10. In a medium-sized bowl stir together the sugar and butter until combined. Add the flour and salt, and mix until combined and crumbly to make the streusel.

11. Evenly add the streusel over each of the muffins, it looks like too much but it's not, use it all.

12. Bake muffins at 425°F for 5 minutes. Then, reduce the heat to 350°F and bake for an additional 16-18 minutes or until a toothpick can be inserted into the center of a muffin and it comes out mostly clean.

13. Let the muffins cool in the tin for 5 minutes then carefully take them out and let them cool completely on a wire rack. Serve warm or at room temperature.

Prep Time: 20 Minutes

Cook Time: 1hrs 15 Minutes

Servings: 8

Ingredients

Bread Batter:

- ½ cup salted butter softened
- ⅔ cup granulated sugar
- 2 eggs
- 1 teaspoon vanilla extract
- 1 teaspoon baking powder
- 1 ½ cups all-purpose flour
- ½ cup greek yogurt
- ¼ cup milk

Apple mixture:

- 2 medium apples we use granny smith (about 2 cups)
- ½ cup brown sugar paked
- 1 teaspoon cinnamon
- Brown Sugar Cinnamon Mixture:

- ¼ cup brown sugar packed
- ½ Tablespoon cinnamon
- 1 teaspoon sugar

Glaze:

- 1 cup powdered sugar
- 3 Tablespoon cream or milk
- 1 teaspoon vanilla extract

Instructions

1. Preheat the oven to 350 degrees. Prepare a 9x5-inch loaf pan by spraying it with non-stick spray.
2. In a large bowl, beat together ½ cup butter and ⅔ cup sugar until smooth.
3. Then, one at a time, beat in the eggs.
4. Mix in 1 teaspoon vanilla extract.
5. Mix in baking powder and flour. Mix only until blended, do not overmix.
6. Add greek yogurt and milk into batter and gently mix just until smooth. Set this aside.
7. In a separate bowl, stir together the apple coating, ½ cup brown sugar and 1 teaspoon cinnamon. Set this aside.
8. Peel and dice the 2 apples. Add these to the brown sugar and cinnamon mixture to coat.

9. In a small bowl mix together the brown sugar cinnamon mixture ¼ cup brown sugar, ½ Tablespoon cinnamon and 1 teaspoon granulated sugar and mix until combined.

10. Pour half of the batter into the prepared loaf pan. Then layer on half the apple mixture.

11. Sprinkle ½ of the brown sugar/cinnamon/sugar mixture on top of the apple layer. Gently swirl a knife through the layers.

12. Then we'll repeat the layers one more time: batter, then apple mixture, then end with the brown sugar-cinnamon mixture. Again, use a knife to swirl through the layers.

13. Bake the loaf until it is fully cooked (you can check by inserting a toothpick, if it comes out clean it's done). Check it after 50 minutes, then after each 5 minutes. I f the loaf starts getting dark on top before fully baked, place a piece of foil over the top to protect it from burning.

14. When the loaf is removed from the oven it needs to cool for at least 30 minutes before you add the glaze (otherwise it will all soak in).

15. While the loaf is cooling, make the glaze. Whisk together powdered sugar, cream, and vanilla until smooth.

16. Pour over bread and serve.

Prep Time: 15 Minutes

Cook Time: 25 Minutes

Servings: 4

Ingredients

For the tortillas:

- ¼ cup vegetable oil
- 6 white corn tortillas cut into bite-sized pieces
- Kosher salt to taste

For assembly:

- 1 small red bell pepper small-diced
- 1 small green bell pepper small-diced
- 1 small sweet onion small diced
- 6 large eggs
- 1 tablespoon whole milk
- ¾ teaspoon kosher salt
- 1/2 teaspoon black pepper
- 10 ounce can diced tomatoes with green chiles drained
- 1 cup shredded Monterey Jack cheese divided

- 1 cup shredded sharp cheddar cheese divided
- ¼ cup fresh chopped cilantro plus more for garnish

Favorite taco toppings

Instructions

1. Over medium heat in a large skillet add the oil.
2. Once the oil is hot, add handfuls of the tortillas and fry them until they're golden brown and crisp. Drain them on a paper-towel-lined sheet tray, and immediately sprinkle with a little salt. Repeat with the rest of the tortillas.
3. Add the red bell pepper, green bell pepper, and onion to the hot skillet over medium-low. Cook everything, stirring occasionally until everything is softened and lightly browned. This typically takes 12-15 minutes.
4. In a medium sized mixing bowl, add the eggs, milk, salt, and pepper, and beat well before setting aside.
5. Add the diced tomatoes with green chiles to the skillet and mix with the peppers and onions.
6. Pour the egg mixture into the skillet and let it cook for one minute. Gently stir until it begins to set up, which typically takes 2-3 minutes.

7. Add half of the shredded Monterey Jack cheese, half of the cheddar, and the cilantro, and stir to combine.

8. Add the fried tortillas to the mixture, stir to combine well.

9. Remove from the heat and sprinkle the remaining cheese on top. Place a lid on top until the cheese is melted.

10. Serve immediately with your favorite taco toppings and enjoy.

Prep Time: 30 Minutes

Cook Time: 15 Minutes

Servings: 32

Ingredients

- 1 large egg
- Splash of water
- 2 sheets puff pastry thawed
- 8 ounces cream cheese softened
- ¾ cup powdered sugar plus more for dusting
- 1 tablespoon vanilla extract
- 2 cups heavy cream
- 1 ½ tablespoons unsweetened cocoa powder

Instructions

1. Preheat the oven to 400°F. Line sheet trays with parchment paper, set aside.
2. Lightly spray cream horn molds with cooking spray, set aside.

3. In a small bowl whisk together the egg and water, set aside.

4. One at a time, unfold one of the puff pastry sheets. Use a rolling pin to flatten it out.

5. Cut the pastry into 8 1-inch sections, and discard any scraps.

6. Starting at the tip of one of the molds, start to wrap a pastry strip around the mold. I like to gently press it together to seal. Place it seam side down onto a prepared sheet tray.

7. Brush the exposed pastry with the egg wash.

8. Bake for 14-16 minutes until puffed and golden brown. Let them cool on the sheet tray in the mold.

9. You will most likely have to bake in batches, so continue to wrap your molds while your batches are baking.

10. Once all of the horns are baked, transfer them to a wire rack to cool completely.

11. While you are waiting for them to cool, make the filling. Place the cream cheese into the body of a stand mixer with the whisk attachment. Whip until smooth.

12. Add the powdered sugar a little at a time until fully mixed in, and scrape down the sides as needed. Stir in the vanilla.

13. Slowly stream in the heavy cream until mixed in. Scrape down the sides, then place the mixer on medium-high speed and whip until stiff peaks form, about 1 minute.

14. Take out half of the cream and place it in a bowl. Add the cocoa powder to the stand mixer and mix it in until combined.

15. Lightly dust the horns with powdered sugar if using.

16. I like to use a pastry bag with an open star tip to fill the cream horns. Fill half of the cream horns with the vanilla cream and the other half with the chocolate cream, and serve immediately.

11. Pizza Grilled Cheese

Prep Time: 10 Minutes

Cook Time: 15 Minutes

Servings: 4

Ingredients

- ½ cup unsalted butter very soft
- 1 tablespoon grated parmesan cheese
- 1 teaspoon garlic powder
- ½ teaspoon dried Italian seasoning
- For assembly:
- 8 slices white bread
- 12 slices mozzarella cheese
- 6 ounces pepperoni
- Warm pizza sauce for dipping

Instructions

1. In a medium-sized bowl, place the butter, parmesan cheese, garlic powder, and Italian seasoning and mix it together until all is combined and smooth.

2. Spread the butter mixture over one side of the bread slices evenly. Then lay the pieces of bread butter side up onto a sheet tray until you're ready to use them.

3. Over medium-low heat, in a skillet, place a piece of bread butter side down into the skillet. Then place a slice of mozzarella on top of the bread. Then, add 6 pepperoni slices, followed by another slice of mozzarella cheese, 6 more pepperonis, and a final slice of mozzarella cheese.

4. Place the top piece of bread on, butter side up. You may end up with leftover pepperoni.

5. Place a lid on the skillet to help melt the cheese, and cook until the bottom of the bottom piece of bread is a golden brown, typically takes about 3-5 minutes. Carefully flip the sandwich over using a spatula. Place the lid back on again and continue to cook the other side, until it's golden brown on the bottom and the cheese is melted in the center. Repeat with the remaining sandwiches.

6. Serve immediately with warm pizza sauce for dipping and enjoy.

Prep Time: 15 Minutes

Cook Time: 20 Minutes

Servings: 4

Ingredients

- 4 hoagie rolls
- ½ cup unsalted butter softened
- 1 tablespoon grated parmesan
- 1 teaspoon garlic powder
- ½ teaspoon Italian seasoning
- 8 slices provolone cheese
- 8 ounces sliced tavern ham
- 4 ounces sliced Genoa salami
- 12 slices deli pepperoni
- ¼ cup sliced pepperoncini peppers

Instructions

1. Preheat the oven to 375F and slice your hoagie rolls in half lengthwise. Do not cut all the way through. Place them cut side open onto a sheet tray.

2. Add the softened butter, parmesan, garlic powder, and Italian seasoning to a small bowl and mix to create a garlic butter.

3. Stir until everything is well combined.

4. Using a knife, spread the garlic butter over the exposed hoagie rolls evenly.

5. Place the buttered rolls in the oven and bake them for 5 minutes or until they're lightly toasted.

6. Cut a piece of cheese in half and place it on the bottom part of the hoagie roll. Repeat with the other rolls.

7. Add ham, salami, and pepperoni, all in top of the cheese- evenly distributed on all of the sandwiches.

8. Add the sliced pepperoncini next. Cut another piece of cheese in half and place it on top of the meat. Repeat the layering of cheese and meat with the rest of the sandwiches.

9. Close the top piece of bread on the sandwiches and place them into a 9x13 baking dish or one similar in size so all the sandwiches fit. Bake them for another 10-15 minutes until the cheese is melted and the sandwiches are warmed through and bread is toasted. Serve immediately and enjoy.

Prep Time: 15 Minutes

Cook Time: 15 Minutes

Servings: 4

Ingredients

For the burger:

- 1 ½ pounds ground beef
- 1 teaspoon garlic powder
- 1 teaspoon onion powder
- 1 teaspoon kosher salt
- ½ teaspoon black pepper

For the gravy:

- 2 cups low sodium beef broth
- 3 tablespoons cornstarch
- 1 beef bullion cube
- 1 teaspoon garlic powder
- 1 teaspoon onion powder
- 1 teaspoon Worcestershire sauce
- 1 tablespoon unsalted butter
- 1 tablespoon heavy cream

For assembly:

- 2 tablespoons unsalted butter
- 4 large eggs
- Salt to taste
- Pepper to taste
- 2 cups hot cooked white rice
- Thinly sliced green onions for garnish

Instructions

1. Mix together the ground beef, garlic powder, onion powder, salt, and pepper in a large mixing bowl. Divide the mixture into fourths and form into patties.
2. Over medium heat, heat a cast iron skillet or large skillet. Add the patties to the heated skillet and sear patty on both sides. Continue to cook burger to your desired temperature, up to 15 minutes total.
3. While the patties are cooking, make the Hawaiian Moco Loco gravy. Whisk together the beef broth, cornstarch, bouillon, garlic powder, onion powder, and Worcestershire sauce in a small saucepan.
4. Place the saucepan over medium heat and cook, stirring occasionally so it doesn't stick or burn. Make sure the bouillon cube breaks up, and cook until the

mixture thickens, which typically takes about 8 minutes. Take it off the heat and stir in the butter and heavy cream, and set aside.

5. Heat a separate nonstick skillet over medium heat. Add the butter to the pan and let it melt. Crack the eggs into the pan and season with salt and pepper to taste. Cook until eggs are sunny side up or over easy, per your preference.

6. To serve, add hot rice to your serving plate. Top with burger patty, add gravy then an egg on top. Garnish with green onions, serve and enjoy.

Prep Time: 15 Minutes

Cook Time: 15 Minutes

Servings: 1

Ingredients

- 3 slices white bread toasted
- Mayonnaise to taste
- 1 slice beefsteak tomato
- Salt and pepper to taste
- 2 slices deli turkey
- 2 slices cheddar cheese
- 2 sliced crispy bacon
- 2 slices deli ham
- 1 leaf green leaf lettuce

Instructions

1. Place one piece of toasted bread on a plate and add desired amount of mayonnaise to the slice.
2. Add 1 slice of a beefsteak tomato on top of the mayo, sprinkle salt and pepper to taste on top of the tomato.

3. Add 2 slices of deli turkey on top of that, followed by 1 piece of sliced cheddar cheese.

4. Break one piece of bacon in half and put it on top of the cheddar cheese.

5. Place another piece of toasted bread on top of the bacon, and smear more mayonnaise to your taste before adding 2 slices of deli ham.

6. Top with 1 slice of green leaf lettuce before breaking the last piece of bacon in half and putting that on top.

7. Smear mayo no the last slice of toast and place it, mayonnaise side down on top of the sandwich.

8. Cut the Club Sandwich into triangles and secure with toothpicks before serving.

Prep Time: 15 Minutes

Cook Time: 15 Minutes

Servings: 4

Ingredients

- 2 pounds boneless skinless chicken breasts
- 3 cloves garlic minced
- 1 Tablespoon apple cider vinegar
- 2 Tablespoons lemon juice
- 1 Tablespoon olive oil
- ½ cup full-fat greek yogurt
- 2 teaspoons oregano
- 2 teaspoons cumin
- 1 teaspoon paprika
- 1 teaspoon salt
- ½ teaspoon pepper
- 1 teaspoon seasoning salt
- 1 teaspoon greek seasoning Cavender's
- 4 pita wraps
- optional toppings: sliced red onion sliced grape tomatoes, shredded lettuce, tzatziki sauce

Instructions

1. Using a meat tenderizer, pound the chicken flat so it's about ¼ inch in thickness.

2. Add all the marinade ingredients, garlic, apple cider vinegar, lemon juice, olive oil, greek yogurt, oregano, cumin, paprika, salt, pepper, seasoning salt, and greek seasoning into a mixing bowl and whisk to combine.

3. Pour the marinade into a large ziptop bag and then add the chicken. Massage everything around to cover every part of the chicken. Put this in the refrigerator for at least 2 hours to marinate, longer is better.

4. Once the chicken has finished marinating, remove the chicken from the marinade and you can toss the rest of the marinade.

5. Place the chicken into a large skillet with a tablespoon of oil.

6. Place heat on medium and cook the chicken for 3-4 minutes, making sure to sear the chicken as it cooks. Then flip the chicken and continue cooking until it's thoroughly cooked or until it reaches an internal temperature of 165 degrees F.

7. Place cooked chicken on a cutting board and let it rest for at least 5 minutes before cutting it up into lengthwise strips.

8. Prep your pita wraps by warming them up slightly so they are nice and pliable before filling them with chicken, toppings, and tzatziki sauce.

Prep Time: 10 Minutes

Cook Time: 10 Minutes

Servings: 8

Ingredients

- 8 hot dogs
- 2 cheddar cheese sticks cut into 4ths by length
- 11 ounce can pizza dough
- 2 eggs
- 2 Tablespoons water
- 2 Tablespoons flaky salt

Nacho Cheese Sauce:

- 2 Tablespoons salted butter
- 1 Tablespoon all-purpose flour
- ½ cup whole milk
- 2 cups shredded cheddar cheese
- 2 Tablespoons cream cheese
- 1 teaspoon black pepper
- 2 teaspoon sriracha

Instructions

1. Cut a slit into the middle of the hot dogs. Add slice of cheese.
2. Cut pizza roll dough into 8 equal sections. Wrap dough around the hot dog, overlapping slightly with each wrap.
3. In a small bowl, whisk eggs and water. Brush hot dogs with egg wash and sprinkle with salt
4. Preheat air fryer to 390* for 5 minutes. Cook pretzel dogs in a single layer with plenty of room in between each one for 7 minutes, flipping halfway through.
5. While pretzel dogs are cooking, make cheese sauce. Create a rouge by melting butter in a saucepan and stirring in flour. Slowly incorporate milk and bring to a boil. Lower heat to a simmer. Add cheese, cream cheese, black pepper, and sriracha. Stir until cheese is melted.
6. Serve immediately with cheese dip and enjoy!

Prep Time: 10 Minutes

Cook Time: 10 Minutes

Servings: 2-4

Ingredients

- 1 cup all-purpose flour
- 1 teaspoon kosher salt
- 1 teaspoon black pepper
- ½ teaspoon garlic powder
- ½ teaspoon onion powder
- 2 large eggs
- 1 tablespoon water
- 1 tablespoon hot sauce
- 1 pound chicken tenderloins
- Olive Oil Spray

Instructions

1. If your air fryer requires preheating, preheat to 400°F.

2. In a medium-sized bowl, whisk together the flour, salt, pepper, garlic powder, and onion powder, set aside.

3. In a medium-sized bowl, whisk together the eggs, water, and hot sauce until fully combined, set aside.

4. One at a time, place the tenders into the flour mixture and coat on all sides, shake off any excess.

5. Place the tender into the egg mixture until fully coated, let any excess egg drip off.

6. Lastly place it back into the flour mixture and pack the flour on the tender to form a crust. Shake off any excess.

7. Spray the air fryer basket with olive oil spray, place the tenders not touching into the basket, you may need to do this in batches.

8. Spray the tops well with more olive oil spray, you want to make sure there are no dry patches.

9. Air fry for 10 minutes, flipping halfway through. After flipping, spray with more olive oil spray.

10. Chicken tenders are ready when they are golden brown and the internal temperature reaches at least 165°F. Serve with your favorite dipping sauce.

Prep Time: 10 Minutes

Cook Time: 10 Minutes

Servings: 4

Ingredients

- 10 ounces canned tuna drained (2 5 ounce cans)
- ⅓ cup mayonnaise
- ¼ cup of red onion diced
- 1 teaspoon lemon juice
- Pinch of salt
- Pinch of pepper
- 1 rib of celery diced
- 1 green onion finely sliced
- 4 slices of cheddar cheese
- 8 slices of tomato
- 8 slices bread
- 2 Tablespoons salted butter softened

Instructions

1. After draining the tuna thoroughly, place it into a medium bowl. Use a fork to break it up well.
2. Mix mayonnaise, onion, lemon juice, salt, pepper, celery, green onion, and green onion with the tuna.
3. Heat a skillet to medium-low heat.
4. Spread butter on one slice of bread. Place this piece of bread, butter side down, into the skillet. Add about ½ cup of the tuna mixture and spread it to the edges of the bread.
5. Add slices of tomato and a slice of cheese.
6. Butter on one side of another piece of bread. Place this piece of bread (butter side up) on top of the cheese. (The butter goes on the outside of the sandwich so that it will toast nicely.) Then carefully flip the sandwich with a spatula to grill both sides.
7. Cook the sandwich in the skillet at medium-low heat until the cheese is melted, and the bread is toasted.

Prep Time: 10 Minutes

Cook Time: 10 Minutes

Servings: 4

Ingredients

- 8 Tablespoons unsalted butter softened
- ¾ cup light brown sugar
- 2 large eggs
- 2 cups mashed bananas about 5 medium bananas
- ½ cup sour cream
- 2 teaspoons ground cinnamon
- 1 teaspoon vanilla extract
- 2 cups all-purpose flour
- ¾ teaspoon baking soda
- ½ teaspoon baking powder
- pinch of fine sea salt

Instructions

1. Preheat the oven to 350°F. Spray a 9x5 loaf pan with baking spray, set aside.

2. Cream together the butter and brown sugar in the body of a stand mixer with the paddle attachment or in a large bowl with an electric hand mixer until light and fluffy, 2 minutes.

3. Add the eggs one at a time, stirring them in completely after each addition. Scrape down the sides.

4. Add the mashed bananas, sour cream, cinnamon, and vanilla, mix it in until combined fully. Scrape down the sides.

5. Lastly, add the flour, baking soda, baking powder, and sea salt into the mixer. Stir together until just combined with no dry patches.

6. Pour the batter into the loaf pan and smooth out the top.

7. Bake for 55-65 minutes until a toothpick inserted into the center comes out clean. At the 20 minute mark, very loosely place a piece of foil on top so the bread doesn't get too brown.

8. Place the pan on a wire rack and let it cool for 10 minutes. Take the bread out of the pan and let it cool completely on the wire rack. Serve warm or room temperature.

Prep Time: 10 Minutes

Cook Time: 10 Minutes

Servings: 4

Ingredients

For the tenders:

- 1 cup all-purpose flour
- 1 teaspoon baking powder
- ½ teaspoon cayenne pepper
- ½ teaspoon garlic powder
- ½ teaspoon kosher salt
- ½ teaspoon black pepper
- ¾ cup buttermilk
- 1 large egg
- 1 pound chicken tenderloins

For the sauce:

- ¼ cup unsalted butter
- 1 ½ tablespoons light brown sugar packed
- ½ teaspoon cayenne pepper
- ½ teaspoon garlic powder

- ½ teaspoon onion powder
- ½ teaspoon kosher salt
- Oil for frying

Instructions

1. In a medium-sized bowl, add the flour, baking powder, cayenne, garlic powder, salt, and pepper, whisk to combine, set aside.
2. In a medium-sized bowl, whisk together the buttermilk and the egg until combined, set aside.
3. Start heating up your oil to 325°F. I like to use a dutch oven for this. You can also use a deep fryer or a large skillet with deep sides. You need about 3 inches of oil up the side of the pan. Make sure you do not overfill the skillet if you are using it, when adding the tenders the oil will rise.
4. While the oil heats, bread the tenders. Do this one tender at a time.
5. Place tender into the flour mixture. Shake off any excess.
6. Place it into the buttermilk mixture and coat the tender well, let any excess drip off.

7. Place it back into the flour mixture, coat the tender in the flour and pat down the flour on the tender so it sticks well and forms a crust. Shake off any excess flour.

8. Next, place the tenders very carefully into the hot oil. Fry for about 3-5 minutes per side, or until the internal temperature reaches 165°F. Place the tenders on a wire rack above a sheet tray while you fry the remaining tenders.

9. Add the butter into a small saucepan over medium-low heat. Let the butter melt then add the brown sugar, cayenne, garlic powder, onion powder, and salt.

10. Whisk to combine and continue to whisk until the sugar dissolves and the sauce comes together for about 2 minutes.

11. Brush the tenders with the sauce and serve.

21. Chicken Sausage & Vegetable Sheet Pan Meal

Prep Time: 10 Minutes

Cook Time: 40 Minutes

Servings: 6

Ingredients

- 1 large zucchini sliced and cut in half
- 1 small head broccoli
- 1 red pepper diced
- 1 yellow pepper diced
- 1 orange pepper diced
- 3/4 lb green beans trimmed and cut in half if needed
- 2 medium red potatoes cut into 1" pieces
- 3 chicken sausage links sliced
- 1/3 cup olive oil
- 2 tsp paprika
- 1 Tbs parsley
- 1 Tbs oregano
- 1 tsp onion powder
- 1 tsp salt
- 1 tsp pepper

- Fresh chopped parsley optional

Instructions

1. Preheat oven to 375.
2. Line a large rimmed baking sheet with tin foil and spray with non-stick cooking spray.
3. Add your vegetables to baking sheet and drizzle with olive oil and stir around to coat.
4. Sprinkle with seasonings and stir around again to coat.
5. Place in oven and bake for 20 minutes, then stir to ensure even cooking.
6. Bake for another 10-20 minutes checking for doneness after 10 minutes.
7. Remove from oven and sprinkle with fresh chopped parsley if desired.

Prep Time: 15 Minutes

Cook Time: 40 Minutes

Servings: 12

Ingredients

For the sauce:

- ½ cup unsalted butter
- ¼ cup all-purpose flour
- 1 tablespoon garlic powder
- 1 teaspoon black pepper
- ½ teaspoon kosher salt
- 1 ½ cups whole milk
- ½ cup unsalted chicken stock
- ½ cup heavy cream
- 8 ounces cream cheese softened and diced
- ½ cup grated parmesan cheese

For assembly:

- 16 ounces penne pasta cooked and drained well
- 3 cups cooked shredded chicken
- 3 cups shredded mozzarella cheese

- Fresh chopped parsley for garnish optional

Instructions

1. Preheat the oven to 375°F. Spray a 9x13 baking dish with cooking spray, and set aside.
2. In a dutch oven or large pot, make the sauce by melting the butter over medium heat. Once melted, whisk in the flour, garlic powder, pepper, and salt, and cook for 1 minute.
3. Slowly stream in the milk while constantly whisking to avoid lumps. Repeat with the chicken stock and heavy cream, the mixture should be smooth.
4. Add the cream cheese and stir it in until melted.
5. Add the parmesan and stir to combine. Take off the heat.
6. Add the cooked penne and shredded chicken to the pot, and stir until everything is coated in the sauce.
7. Pour half the mixture into the prepared baking dish, and top with half of the mozzarella cheese.
8. Add the remaining pasta on top, followed by the remaining mozzarella.

9. Bake uncovered for 20 minutes until bubbly. Turn on the broiler and broil until golden brown. Serve immediately with parsley garnish if desired.

Prep Time: 15 Minutes

Cook Time: 1hrs 40 Minutes

Servings: 16

Ingredients

For the potatoes:

- 8 small russet potatoes
- 1 tablespoon olive oil
- 2 teaspoons kosher salt
- For the potato skins:
- 3 tablespoons salted butter melted
- ½ teaspoon black pepper
- ¼ teaspoon garlic powder
- ¼ teaspoon onion powder
- ¼ teaspoon smoked paprika

For the filling:

- 8 ounces shredded sharp cheddar cheese
- 8 slices bacon cooked crispy and crumbled
- Sour cream to serve
- Thinly sliced green onions to serve

Instructions

1. Preheat the oven to 400°F. Wash the potatoes very well and pat them dry with a paper towel, place them on a sheet tray.

2. Using a fork, pierce the potatoes all over so any excess steam can escape.

3. Brush the outsides with the olive oil, then sprinkle with the salt all over.

4. Bake for 30-60 minutes, depending on the size of the potatoes, until a knife inserted into the potatoes goes in smoothly. Let them cool completely, or until they are cool enough to handle on the sheet tray.

5. In a small bowl, stir together the melted butter, pepper, garlic powder, onion powder, and smoked paprika.

6. Cut the potatoes in half and scoop out the insides, leaving about ¼ inch of the potato attached to the skin.

7. Place them cut side down onto the sheet tray and brush the outside with half of the butter mixture.

8. Bake for 8 minutes, turn them over, and brush the inside of the potatoes with the remaining butter mixture. Bake an additional 8 minutes until the edges are golden brown and crispy.

9. Add the cheese and bacon evenly to the inside cup of
    the potato skins.

10. Bake an additional 5 minutes until the cheese is
    melted. Serve immediately with sour cream and
    scallions.

Prep Time: 15 Minutes

Cook Time: 1hrs 20 Minutes

Servings: 12

Ingredients

- 12 cups white bread cubes ½-inch diced
- 1 cup + 4 tablespoons unsalted butter divided
- 1 ½ cups chopped celery
- 1 ½ cups chopped onion
- 4 cloves garlic minced
- 1 tablespoon dried parsley flakes
- 2 teaspoons kosher salt
- 2 teaspoons ground sage
- 1 ½ teaspoons black pepper
- 1 teaspoon dried thyme
- 1 teaspoon poultry seasoning
- ½ teaspoon dried rosemary
- 2 large eggs well beaten
- 2-3 cups unsalted chicken stock
- Fresh chopped parsley for garnish

Instructions

1. Let the bread cubes sit out overnight if you have time. If not, bake them in a single layer on sheet trays at 200°F for 30 minutes, stirring every 10 minutes. Set aside.

2. Spray an 11x7 baking dish with cooking spray, set aside.

3. In a large skillet over medium heat, melt the 1 cup of the butter. Add the celery and onion, and cook, until softened and the onion is translucent, occasionally stirring for 10 minutes.

4. Add the garlic, parsley, salt, sage, pepper, thyme, poultry seasoning, and rosemary. Mix them in and cook for 1 minute, take off the heat.

5. Mix the eggs and 2 cups of stock together well in a bowl.

6. Add the bread cubes and vegetable mixture to a large bowl, and stir to combine.

7. Add the egg and stock mixture, stir to combine. Let it sit for 10 minutes so the bread can absorb the liquid. It should be very moist but not wet, if it seems too dry to you, add another cup of stock.

8. Pour the stuffing into the prepared baking dish. Melt the remaining 4 tablespoons of butter and drizzle it on top.

9. Cover with foil and bake for 40 minutes. Remove the foil and bake for an additional 20-30 minutes until golden brown and crispy on top. Place a sheet tray under the baking dish to catch any drips.

10. Let cool for 10 minutes and serve with fresh chopped parsley for optional garnish.

Prep Time: 15 Minutes

Cook Time: 30 Minutes

Servings: 15

Ingredients

For the cake:

- 8 ounces pitted dates roughly chopped
- 1 cup boiling water
- 2 cups all-purpose flour
- 1 ½ teaspoons baking powder
- 1 ½ teaspoons baking soda
- ½ teaspoon fine sea salt
- ½ cup unsalted butter softened
- ½ cup demerara sugar
- ½ cup dark brown sugar packed
- 3 large eggs room temp

For the sauce:

- ½ cup unsalted butter
- 2 ¼ cups heavy cream
- 3 cups dark brown sugar packed

- ½ teaspoon fine sea salt
- 1 tablespoon vanilla extract
- Whipped cream to serve optional

Instructions

1. Preheat the oven to 350°F. Spray a 9x13 baking dish with cooking spray, set aside.
2. Place the chopped dates into boiling water and take off the heat. Stir the dates into the water, let them soak for 15 minutes.
3. While the dates soak, make the cake batter. Stir together the flour, baking powder, baking soda, and salt in a medium-sized bowl, set aside.
4. In a large bowl with an electric hand mixer, cream together the butter, demerara sugar, and brown sugar for 3 minutes.
5. Add the eggs one at a time, mixing the first one in before adding the next.
6. Add the dry ingredients and stir to combine, scrape the sides as needed.
7. When the dates are done soaking, use an immersion blender and blend until smooth.
8. Add to the cake batter and mix it in fully.

9. Add the batter to the prepared baking dish and smooth it out. Bake for 25-30 minutes until dark golden brown and a toothpick inserted into the center comes out clean.

10. While the cake is baking, make the sauce. Add the butter to a medium-sized saucepan and melt it over medium-low heat. Add the heavy cream, brown sugar, and salt, and whisk to combine.

11. Continue to whisk occasionally until it comes to a simmer. As soon as it begins to simmer, continuously stir for 2 minutes. Take off the heat and stir in the vanilla, set aside.

12. When the cake comes out of the oven, take a fork and poke holes all over it.

13. Pour half of the sauce all over the cake. Let it sit for 15 minutes to absorb the sauce.

14. Place the broiler on high, and move an oven rack to the second position under the broiler. Place the cake under the broiler and broil for 1-2 minutes until it becomes sticky and bubbly. Make sure to watch it closely, so it doesn't burn. We are not looking to get any color on the cake, just to caramelize the sauce on top.

15. You can serve the cake now, let it cool more, or let it cool completely before serving. Serve with more sauce over each slice and whipped cream if desired.

Prep Time: 15 Minutes

Cook Time: 1hrs 30 Minutes

Servings: 8

Ingredients

For the topping:

- 2 pounds russet potatoes peeled, 1-inch dice
- 8 tablespoons salted butter
- ½ cup whole milk
- ½ cup grated parmesan cheese
- 1 teaspoon kosher salt
- 1 teaspoon black pepper

For the filling:

- 2 tablespoons unsalted butter
- 1 pound lean ground beef
- 1 small sweet onion small diced
- 3 cloves garlic minced
- 1 teaspoon garlic powder
- 1 teaspoon onion powder
- 1 teaspoon kosher salt

- 1 teaspoon black pepper
- 2 tablespoons all-purpose flour
- 1 cup beef stock
- 2 teaspoons Worcestershire sauce
- 12 ounces mixed frozen veggies
- Fresh chopped parsley for garnish optional

Instructions

1. Preheat the oven to 375°F. Add the diced potatoes to a large pot and cover them plus two inches with cold water. Cover, bring to a boil, and boil for about 15 minutes or until the potatoes are fork tender.
2. Drain the potatoes and let them sit in the cooking pot uncovered for 10 minutes to allow excess steam to escape.
3. Add the butter, milk, cheese, salt, and pepper.
4. Mash until smooth.
5. While the potatoes are cooking, make the filling. In a large skillet over medium heat, melt the butter, then brown the ground beef, breaking it up into crumbles until there is no pink left. 10 minutes.
6. Add the onions and continue to cook until softened and translucent, occasionally stirring for 10 minutes.

7. Add the garlic, garlic powder, onion powder, salt, and pepper. Stir everything together and cook for 30 seconds.

8. Add the flour, stir and cook for 1 minute.

9. Next, add the stock and Worcestershire sauce, stir to combine.

10. Add the frozen veggies and mix them in, bring the mixture to a simmer then take off the heat.

11. Add the filling to a 9x13 baking dish in an even layer.

12. Top with the mashed potatoes and smooth out the top.

13. Bake for 40-45 minutes until dark golden brown on top and bubbly. Let cool for 15 minutes, then serve with parsley if using.

Prep Time: 20 Minutes

Cook Time: 3hrs 30 Minutes

Servings: 2

Ingredients

For the sausage:

- ½ pound ground pork
- 2 cloves garlic minced
- 1 ½ teaspoons fennel seeds crushed
- ¼ teaspoon dried basil
- ¼ teaspoon dried oregano
- ¼ teaspoon kosher salt
- ¼ teaspoon black pepper

For the sauce:

- 14 ounces crushed tomatoes
- 1 tablespoon grated parmesan cheese
- 1 ½ teaspoons dried basil
- 1 ½ teaspoons dried oregano
- ½ teaspoon garlic powder
- ½ teaspoon onion powder

- For assembly:

- 1 pound pizza dough thawed

- 8 ounces sliced mozzarella cheese

- 2 tablespoons grated parmesan plus more for serving

- Drizzle of olive oil

- Fresh chopped parsley optional

Instructions

1. In a medium-sized bowl, mix together the ground pork, garlic, fennel, dried basil, dried oregano, salt, and pepper.

2. Place a skillet over medium-high heat. Once hot, add the sausage and break it up into crumbles, cooking it until cooked through and there is no pink left. Let it drain on paper towels.

3. In a medium-sized bowl, stir together the crushed tomatoes, parmesan, dried basil, dried oregano, garlic powder, and onion powder.

4. Place a large piece of parchment paper on your work surface. Place the pizza dough in the center. Stretch it out to an oval shape or the shape of your 8-quart slow cooker.

5. Lift the pizza dough up using the parchment paper to help and place it in the slow cooker. If you have to adjust it more in the slow cooker, do so now.

6. Press the mozzarella into the dough, leaving a ½-inch border. Add the cooked sausage on top, followed by the pizza sauce. Add the 2 tablespoons of parmesan and finally a drizzle of olive oil.

7. Carefully lift the edges of the crust, so it sits above the fillings.

8. Place a large piece of paper towel over the slow cooker and put the lid on. Place on high for 2-3 hours or low 4-5 hours.

9. Lift the pizza out by the parchment once it is done and let it sit for 15 minutes. Slice and serve with more parmesan and fresh chopped parsley if desired.

Prep Time: 20 Minutes

Cook Time: 10 Minutes

Servings: 4

Ingredients

- 2 pounds ribeye steak
- 1 ½ cups all-purpose flour
- 1 ½ teaspoons baking powder
- ¾ teaspoon baking soda
- ¾ teaspoon kosher salt
- ¾ teaspoon black pepper
- ¾ teaspoon garlic powder
- ¾ cup buttermilk
- 1 large egg
- 1 tablespoon hot sauce
- Peanut oil for frying

For the gravy:

- ¼ cup reserved cooking oil
- ⅓ cup all-purpose flour
- 2 cups whole milk

- ½ teaspoon kosher salt
- ½ teaspoon black pepper

Instructions

1. Cut the steak into ½-inch strips, and remove any fat you don't want.
2. In a shallow bowl, stir together the flour, baking powder, baking soda, salt, pepper, and garlic powder.
3. In another shallow bowl, whisk together the buttermilk, egg, and hot sauce.
4. Take a handful of the steak strips at a time and place them into the flour mixture, and coat them in the flour.
5. Shake off any excess and dip them into the egg mixture, letting excess drip off.
6. Last, place them back into the flour mixture and coat them well. Gently press the flour into the strips, so it sticks.
7. Place the strips, not touching on a parchment-lined sheet tray while you coat the remaining steak strips.
8. Add 1/4th inch of peanut oil to a cast iron or heavy bottom skillet. Heat until the oil reaches 325°F over medium heat.

9. Carefully add the steak strips to the pan and fry them for 5 minutes, flipping them halfway through. We are looking for them to be golden brown and crispy.

10. Take out the steak strips with tongs and place them on a wire rack set on a sheet tray to catch any drips. Repeat with the remaining steak strips.

11. Pour out any excess oil from the pan, leaving about ¼ cup in the skillet. Add the flour and whisk it into the oil. Cook for 1 minute.

12. Slowly stream in the milk while whisking constantly.

13. Season with the salt and pepper.

14. Continuing to whisk, bring to a simmer and simmer until thickened. Serve immediately with the steak fingers as a dipping sauce.

Prep Time: 30 Minutes

Cook Time: 30 Minutes

Servings: 4

Ingredients

- 1 pound flank steak
- 2 Tablespoons soy sauce
- 2 Tablespoons cornstarch
- 2 Tablespoons cooking oil
- 2 cups broccoli florets
- 1 cup shredded carrots
- 1 cup snow peas
- 1 red bell pepper sliced
- 1 green onion sliced

Sauce:

- ½ cup soy sauce
- 3 Tablespoons brown sugar
- ½ teaspoon garlic powder
- 1 teaspoon ginger
- 2 Tablespoons sesame seeds toasted

Instructions

1. Cut beef thinly across the grain (no more than ½ inch thick, 2-inch-long strips). Place it in a freezer bag (or medium bowl). Stir in 2 Tablespoons of soy sauce and the 2 Tablespoons cornstarch and set aside. Allow this to marinate at room temperature for at least 30 minutes.
2. Prepare the vegetables and set aside.
3. Prepare the sauce: Whisk together ½ cup soy sauce, brown sugar, garlic powder, and ginger. Set this aside.
4. Heat the oil to high heat in a large deep skillet or wok. Add half of the meat to the skillet and fry for 3 minutes. Remove this meat from the skillet and fry the other half. Then remove it from the skillet. (You don't want to crowd the meat, or it will not sear properly.)
5. Add the vegetables (except the green onions) to the skillet and fry for 2 minutes.
6. Then add the beef back to the skillet. Stir in the sauce and heat through.
7. Sprinkle the green onions and toasted sesame seeds over top.
8. Serve with noodles or rice.

Prep Time: 30 Minutes

Cook Time: 1hrs 30 Minutes

Servings: 12

Ingredients

For the meat:

- 1 ½ pounds lean ground beef
- 1 pound ground Italian sausage
- 2 teaspoons garlic powder
- 2 teaspoons onion powder
- ½ cup grated parmesan cheese
- ¼ teaspoon kosher salt
- ¼ teaspoon black pepper

For the sauce:

- 28 ounces canned whole tomatoes
- 6 garlic cloves minced
- ⅓ cup dry red wine
- 6 ounces tomato paste
- 30 ounces canned tomato sauce
- ½ cup grated parmesan cheese

- 1 ½ tablespoons dried oregano
- 1 ½ tablespoons garlic powder
- 1 ½ tablespoons onion powder
- 1 teaspoon black pepper
- salt to taste

For assembly:

- 1 pound lasagna noodles
- 15 ounces ricotta cheese
- 1 large egg
- ¼ cup parmesan cheese
- 6 cups shredded mozzarella cheese
- ½ teaspoon dried oregano
- ¼ teaspoon garlic powder
- Fresh chopped basil for garnish optional
- Fresh chopped parsley for garnish optional

Instructions

1. In a large bowl add the ground beef, sausage, garlic powder, onion powder, parmesan cheese, salt, and pepper. Mix together until combined.

2. Heat a dutch oven or large pot over medium-high heat. Add the meat mixture and brown it, breaking it

up into crumbles until no longer pink, 10-15 minutes. Drain any excess liquid that comes off the meat.

3. While the meat is cooking, put the whole tomatoes into a large bowl along with the juice. Using your hands, crush the tomatoes into small pieces, discard any hard pieces of tomato, set aside.

4. Add the minced garlic cloves to the pot and mix them in, cook until fragrant, 30 seconds. Add the wine and tomato paste, mix it in. If there are any browned bits on the bottom of the pan, scrape them off.

5. Add the tomatoes you crushed by hand along with the tomato sauce, parmesan, oregano, garlic powder, onion powder, and black pepper. Mix it in fully until combined.

6. Bring to a boil, reduce heat to a simmer, cover and simmer for at least 30 minutes. If you can let it simmer longer, I suggest you do, up to 2 more hours. Stirring occasionally.

7. Taste the sauce and add more salt or other seasonings if needed to your taste.

8. While the sauce is simmering, cook the lasagna noodles per the directions on the back of the box. Drain them.

9. Spray a large sheet tray lightly with cooking spray. Lay the noodles out flat, spraying the tops lightly with more cooking spray between layers so they don't stick together.

10. Preheat the oven to 375°F. Spray a 9x13x3 baking dish with cooking spray, set aside.

11. In a medium-sized bowl, stir together the ricotta, egg, parmesan, and half of the mozzarella set aside.

12. To assemble the lasagna, spread a heaping cup of the sauce on the bottom of the baking dish.

13. Place 4 lasagna noodles down the length of the dish, they will need to overlap a little to fit.

14. Spread ⅓ of the cheese mixture on top of the noodles.

15. Spread another heaping cup of the sauce on top.

16. Repeat two more times with the noodles, cheese mixture, and sauce with another layer of noodles on top. You may not use all of the lasagna noodles. Top the whole thing with 1 & ½ cups of the sauce. Cover with foil.

17. Bake for 25 minutes until bubbly. Take off the foil and add the remaining cheese. Sprinkle the dried oregano and garlic powder on top. Place it back in the oven and bake for 5-8 more minutes until the cheese is melted.

18. If you want to brown the cheese, turn the broiler on high and broil until you reach your desired browning. Make sure to watch it the entire time so it doesn't burn.

19. Take out of the oven and let it sit for 15 minutes before slicing to serve. Garnish with fresh chopped basil and parsley if desired.